PILATES BAR WORKOUTS FOR BEGINNERS

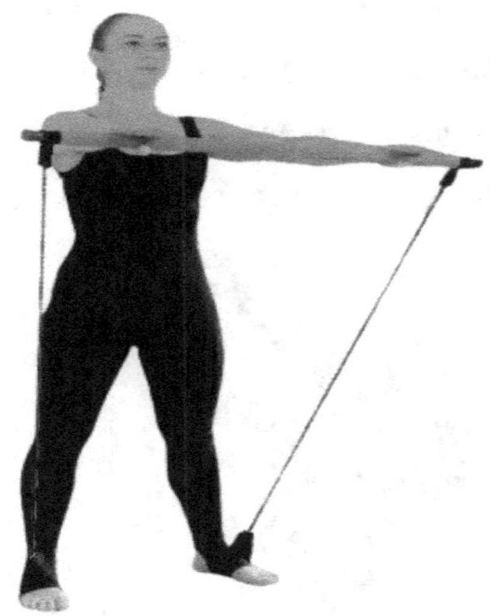

The Easy Step By Step Guide For Men And Women To Lose Weight, Prevent Aging And Enhance Mobility, Strength, Flexibility And Balance With Simple Daily Exercises

Randy T. Lucas

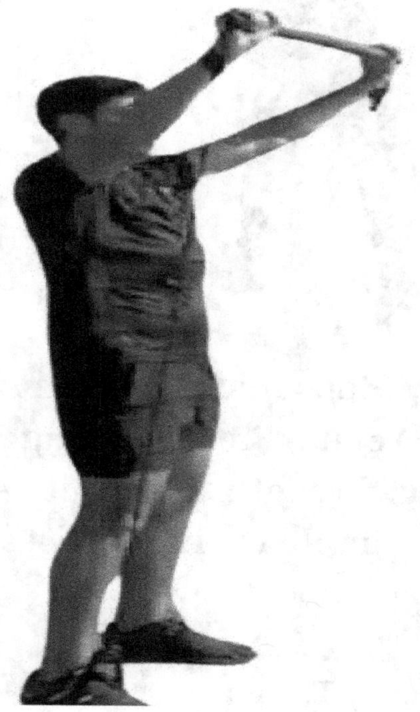

Table of Contents

INTRODUCTION

In the heart of a bustling city lived Anna, a person whose life was transformed by the grace and strength found in Pilates bar workouts. Once struggling with the demands of a sedentary job and the toll it took on her body and spirit, Anna discovered a path to rejuvenation and empowerment. Her journey from stiffness and discomfort to flexibility, strength, and inner calm exemplifies the transformative power of Pilates bar exercises for beginners. This guide is inspired by stories like Anna's, tailored to introduce you to the world of Pilates bar workouts with clarity and purpose.

"Pilates Bar Workouts for Beginners" is more than just a book; it is a doorway to a healthier, more vibrant version of yourself. Designed with the absolute beginner in mind, this guide demystifies the practice of Pilates bar workouts, making it accessible to all. Whether you're looking to enhance your physical fitness, improve your posture, or find a new source of mental calmness, this book is your starting point.

Within these pages, you'll find a comprehensive introduction to the principles of Pilates, the benefits of incorporating a Pilates bar into your routine, and step-by-step instructions for exercises that are specifically chosen for their efficacy and safety for beginners. Each exercise is designed to build strength, improve flexibility, and increase endurance in a balanced and gentle manner. Furthermore, we emphasize the importance of alignment and breath, core components of Pilates that turn physical movements into a meditative practice.

This book not only guides you through the technical aspects of Pilates bar workouts but also inspires you to embrace this practice as a journey toward holistic well-being. By the end of this guide, you will not only have a solid foundation in Pilates bar exercises but also experience firsthand the transformative effects on your body and mind, much like Anna did. Welcome to the beginning of your Pilates journey—a path to strength, flexibility, and peace.

CHAPTER 1

Understanding Pilates Bar Workouts For Beginners

Understanding Pilates bar workouts for beginners involves recognizing the foundational principles of Pilates which are control, concentration, centering, flow, precision, and breath, and applying them using the Pilates bar as a versatile tool to enhance the workout. This unique piece of equipment adds resistance, assists alignment, and increases the effectiveness of traditional Pilates exercises, making it an excellent choice for those new to the practice. Beginners should approach Pilates bar workouts with an emphasis on mastering form and technique over speed or intensity. The Pilates bar can help stabilize movements, allowing for a deeper connection to the core muscles and facilitating a more focused and mindful exercise session.

For those starting out, it's crucial to learn the correct setup and use of the Pilates bar, understanding how it can be incorporated into exercises to target different muscle groups, improve flexibility, and build strength. It's also important to adapt exercises to individual fitness levels, using modifications suggested by instructors to ensure safety and effectiveness. Embracing Pilates bar workouts opens up a path to improved physical health, offering a balanced approach to strength and flexibility training, with the added benefits of enhancing mental well-being through focused, mindful practice.

Benefits Of Pilates Bar Workouts

1. Improved Flexibility: Pilates bar exercises emphasize smooth, controlled movements that stretch and lengthen the muscles. Over time, this increases joint mobility and muscle elasticity, contributing to an overall improvement in flexibility.

2. Increased Core Strength: At the heart of Pilates is the focus on core strength. The Pilates bar acts as a resistance tool that enhances traditional Pilates exercises, engaging and strengthening the deep abdominal muscles, back, and pelvic floor. This leads to better core stability and strength.

3. Enhanced Posture: Regular Pilates bar workouts strengthen the postural muscles, teaching the body to maintain alignment. This not only improves posture but also reduces the risk of injury and relieves chronic back pain.

4. Low Impact: Ideal for beginners, those with joint issues, or anyone looking for a gentle workout, Pilates bar exercises are low impact. They offer an effective way to build strength and flexibility without putting undue stress on the joints.

5. Increased Mind-Body Connection: Pilates requires concentration and focus as you move through the exercises, paying attention to your breathing and how your body feels. This practice enhances the connection between mind and body, promoting mental clarity and mindfulness.

6. Improved Balance and Coordination: By focusing on controlled movements and core strength, Pilates bar workouts improve balance and coordination. This is particularly beneficial for aging populations and those looking to enhance athletic performance.

7. Weight Management: While Pilates bar workouts are not high intensity, they can still contribute to weight management and body shaping. By building lean muscle mass, the body becomes more efficient at burning calories, even at rest.

8. Increased Energy Levels: Regular participation in Pilates bar workouts can lead to increased energy levels. The focus on breathing and efficient movement patterns helps improve cardiovascular health and stamina.

9. Injury Prevention: Strengthening the body's core and improving flexibility and posture through Pilates bar workouts can significantly reduce the risk of injury. Strong, flexible muscles are less likely to be injured during daily activities or other forms of exercise.

10. Adaptability: Pilates bar workouts are highly adaptable. They can be modified to meet the needs of beginners or those with specific physical challenges, making Pilates an inclusive practice for improving fitness and health.

Safety Precautions And Guidelines

1. Consult a Healthcare Provider: Before starting any new exercise regimen, including Pilates bar workouts, it's advisable to consult with a healthcare provider, especially if you have any pre-existing health conditions or concerns.

2. Start with a Warm-up: Begin each session with a warm-up to prepare your body for exercise. A warm-up can include gentle stretching and movements that mimic the workout to come, increasing blood flow to the muscles and reducing the risk of injury.

3. Use Proper Equipment: Ensure that your Pilates bar and any associated equipment are in good condition. The Pilates bar should be sturdy and able to withstand the exercises without bending or breaking.

4. Focus on Form: Pilates emphasizes precise movements and form. Pay careful attention to your instructor's guidance on alignment and technique to maximize the benefits of each exercise and avoid strain or injury.

5. Pace Yourself: As a beginner, it's important to pace yourself and not rush through the exercises. Performing movements slowly and with control is more beneficial and safer than trying to speed through them.

6. Listen to Your Body: Be attuned to your body's signals. If you feel pain (beyond the normal discomfort of exercising new muscles), stop and assess. Pain can indicate improper form or that a particular exercise is not suitable for you at this time.

7. Stay Hydrated: Drink water before, during, and after your workout to stay hydrated. Proper hydration helps maintain energy levels and aids in muscle recovery.

8. Breathe Properly: Pilates exercises are synchronized with specific breathing patterns. Focusing on your breath not only enhances the effectiveness of the exercises but also prevents strain by ensuring a continuous flow of oxygen to your muscles.

9. Avoid Overexertion: While it's important to challenge yourself, avoid overexertion, which can lead to injury. If you're unable to maintain form or complete an exercise without pain, it's a sign to reduce the intensity or duration of your workout.

10. Seek Professional Guidance: For beginners, working with a certified Pilates instructor can provide valuable insights into proper form, technique, and progression. An instructor can also help modify exercises to suit your fitness level and goals.

WARM UP EXERCISES

1. Arm Circles with Pilates Bar

- **Starting Position:** Position your feet hip-width apart, holding the Pilates bar horizontally in front of you with both hands, arms extended at shoulder height.

- **Steps:** Slowly rotate your arms in forward circles, gradually increasing the size of the circles. After 10 repetitions, reverse the direction for backward circles.

- **Repetitions:** 10 forward, 10 backward.

- **Purpose:** This exercise warms up the shoulders, arms, and upper back, improving mobility and preparing the muscles for exercise.

2. Pilates Bar Squats

- **Starting Position:** Stand with feet slightly wider than hip-width apart, holding the Pilates bar at your chest with both hands.

- **Steps:** Lower into a squat, keeping your back straight and chest lifted, as if sitting back into a chair. Ensure your knees do not extend past your toes. Return to standing.

- **Repetitions:** 10-15.

- **Purpose:** Activates the legs, glutes, and core, while also warming up the spine and improving lower body mobility.

3. Roll Downs

- **Starting Position:** Stand tall with feet hip-width apart, holding the Pilates bar in front of you at hip level.

- **Steps:** Inhale to prepare. As you exhale, tuck your chin to your chest and slowly roll down towards the floor, vertebra by vertebra, allowing the Pilates bar to guide your hands towards the ground. Breathe in at the bottom and out as you steadily raise yourself back up to standing.

- **Repetitions:** 5-8.

- **Purpose:** Increases spinal flexibility, gently stretches the back and hamstrings, and activates the core.

4. Pilates Bar Leg Swings

- **Starting Position:** Stand side-on to a support (e.g., a wall or chair) for balance, holding the support with one hand and the Pilates bar horizontally in front of you with the other hand.

- **Steps:** Swing the leg closest to the support forward and backward in a controlled motion, keeping the Pilates bar stable in front of you.

- **Repetitions:** 10 swings each leg.

- **Purpose:** Loosens the hip joints, warms up the leg muscles, and improves dynamic flexibility and balance.

5. Pilates Bar Chest Expansion

- **Starting Position:** Position your feet hip-width apart and grasp the Pilates bar with both hands while keeping your arms straight.

- **Steps:** Gently press the bar down and away, lifting your chest and squeezing your shoulder blades together. Hold for a moment, then release.

- **Repetitions:** 10-12.

- **Purpose:** Opens up the chest and shoulders, improving posture and breathing capacity, and preparing the upper body for exercise.

CHAPTER 2

WORKOUTS

1. Pilates Bar Presses

- **Starting Position:** Sit on the floor with legs extended in front of you. Hold the Pilates bar with both hands, arms extended at chest level.

- **Steps:** Engage your core and press the bar forward, extending your arms fully. Then, slowly draw the bar back towards your chest.

- **Repetitions:** 10-15.

- **Purpose:** Strengthens the shoulders, chest, and arms, while engaging the core to maintain stability.

2. Standing Pilates Bar Roll-Up

- **Starting Position:** Position your feet hip-width apart, holding the Pilates bar overhead with both hands, arms extended.

- **Steps:** Inhale to prepare. As you exhale, slowly roll down towards your toes, keeping your arms extended and the bar over your head. Inhale at the bottom, then exhale as you slowly roll back up to standing, lifting the bar overhead.

- **Repetitions:** 8-10.

- **Purpose:** Improves spinal flexibility, engages the core, and stretches the hamstrings.

3. Pilates Bar Footwork

- **Starting Position:** Place your feet flat on the floor and bend your knees while lying on your back., hip-width apart. Place the middle of the Pilates bar on the soles of your feet, holding each end with your hands.

- **Steps:** Press your feet against the bar, extending your legs fully. Ensure your core is engaged and your lower back remains in contact with the floor. Slowly return to the starting position.

- **Repetitions:** 10-12.

- **Purpose:** Strengthens the legs and core, while promoting pelvic stability.

4. Pilates Bar Arm Circles

- **Starting Position:** Place your feet flat on the floor and bend your knees while lying on your back. Hold the Pilates bar above your chest with arms extended.

- **Steps:** Keeping your arms straight, slowly circle the bar over your head and then down towards your hips, creating a large circle. Keep your core engaged and lower back pressed into the floor.

- **Repetitions:** 8 circles in each direction.

- **Purpose:** Enhances shoulder mobility and stability, engages the core, and strengthens the arm muscles.

5. Pilates Bar Russian Twists

- **Starting Position:** Sit on the floor with knees bent, feet lifted slightly off the ground. Grasp the Pilates bar at chest height with both hands in front of you.

- **Steps:** Engage your core and rotate your torso to the right, bringing the bar towards the floor beside you. Return to center and then rotate to the left. Keep your feet elevated and steady throughout the movement.

- **Repetitions:** 10-15 on each side.

- **Purpose:** Strengthens the obliques and abdominal muscles, improves rotational mobility, and enhances core stability.

6. Bridge with Pilates Bar

- **Starting Position:** Place your feet flat on the floor and bend your knees while lying on your back., hip-width apart. Hold the Pilates bar with both hands, arms extended towards the ceiling directly above your shoulders.

- **Steps:** Engage your core and lift your hips off the floor into a bridge position, pressing the Pilates bar towards the ceiling. Ensure your shoulders and arms remain steady. Slowly lower your hips back to the starting position.

- **Repetitions:** 10-15.

- **Purpose:** Strengthens the glutes, hamstrings, and core. This exercise also stabilizes the shoulders due to the overhead position of the Pilates bar.

7. Pilates Bar Lunges

- **Starting Position:** Position your feet hip-width apart, holding the Pilates bar in front of you at chest height with both hands.

- **Steps:** Step one foot back into a lunge, bending both knees to about 90 degrees, keeping the Pilates bar steady at chest level. Push through your front heel to return to the starting position. Alternate legs.

- **Repetitions:** 10 on each leg.

- **Purpose:** Builds leg and glute strength, improves balance and stability, and engages the core to maintain posture.

8. Side-Lying Leg Lifts with Pilates Bar

- **Starting Position:** Lie on one side with legs extended, using one hand for support. Place the Pilates bar on the upper side of your top leg, holding it in place at both ends.

- **Steps:** Keeping the bar steady, lift your top leg towards the ceiling then lower it back down with control. Keep your movements slow and focused.

- **Repetitions:** 10-15 on each side.

- **Purpose:** Targets the outer thighs and hips, improves lateral stability, and engages the core muscles for balance.

9. Pilates Bar Plank

- **Starting Position:** Start in a high plank position with hands shoulder-width apart, holding the Pilates bar under your hands on the floor.

- **Steps:** Ensure your body forms a straight line from your head to your heels. Hold this position, keeping the core engaged and the Pilates bar stable under your hands.

- **Repetitions:** Hold for 30-60 seconds.

- **Purpose:** Strengthens the entire core, arms, and shoulders, while improving overall body stability and endurance.

10. Seated Twist with Pilates Bar

- **Starting Position:** Sit with legs extended in front of you, a slight bend in the knees. Hold the Pilates bar horizontally in front of you with both hands.

- **Steps:** Lean back slightly, engaging your core. Rotate your torso to one side, bringing the Pilates bar towards the floor beside you. Return to center and then rotate to the opposite side.

- **Repetitions:** 10-15 on each side.

- **Purpose:** Primarily targets the oblique muscles, enhances spinal rotation mobility, and engages the deep core muscles for stability.

11. Pilates Bar Pull-Overs

- **Starting Position:** Place your feet flat on the floor and bend your knees while lying on your back. Hold the Pilates bar with both hands, arms extended directly above your chest.

- **Steps:** Keeping your arms straight, slowly lower the bar back over your head towards the floor, only as far as comfortable while keeping your lower back pressed into the floor. Bring the bar back to the starting position above your chest.

- **Repetitions:** 10-12.

- **Purpose:** Strengthens the upper back, shoulders, and arms, while engaging the core to maintain stability.

12. Pilates Bar Single-Leg Circles

- **Starting Position:** Lie on your back with one leg extended upwards, foot resting in the center of the Pilates bar, and the other leg flat on the ground. Hold the ends of the bar with both hands to keep it steady.

- **Steps:** Rotate the lifted leg in small circles in the air, keeping the rest of your body still and the Pilates bar stable. Perform circles in both clockwise and counterclockwise directions.

- **Repetitions:** 5-8 circles in each direction per leg.

- **Purpose:** Improves hip mobility and flexibility, strengthens leg muscles, and engages the core for stability.

13. Pilates Bar Bicep Curls

- **Starting Position:** Position your feet hip-width apart, holding the Pilates bar with both hands in front of you, palms facing up.

- **Steps:** Keeping your elbows close to your body, curl the bar up towards your shoulders by bending your elbows. Lower back down with control.

- **Repetitions:** 10-15.

- **Purpose:** Targets the biceps and improves arm strength, while engaging the core to maintain good posture.

14. Pilates Bar Standing Side Bend

- **Starting Position:** Stand with feet slightly wider than hip-width apart, holding the Pilates bar overhead with both hands, arms extended.

- **Steps:** Keeping your hips and shoulders facing forward, bend at the waist to one side as far as comfortable, feeling a stretch along the opposite side. Return to the center and repeat on the other side.

- **Repetitions:** 8-10 on each side.

- **Purpose:** Increases lateral flexibility of the spine, strengthens the obliques and core, and improves posture and balance.

15. Pilates Bar Tricep Dips

- **Starting Position:** Bend your knees and place your feet flat on the floor as you sit on the floor, holding the Pilates bar behind you with both hands, palms facing down.

- **Steps:** Lift your hips off the floor, using your arms to support your weight. Bend your elbows to lower your body towards the floor, then straighten your arms to lift your body back up.

- **Repetitions:** 8-10.

- **Purpose:** Strengthens the triceps and shoulders, enhances core stability, and improves upper body strength.

16. Pilates Bar Toe Taps

- **Starting Position:** Lie on your back with your knees bent into a tabletop position (knees aligned over hips, shins parallel to the floor), holding the Pilates bar above your chest with arms extended.

- **Steps:** Inhale to prepare. As you exhale, lower one foot to tap the floor gently, keeping the other leg stationary and the Pilates bar stable. Inhale to lift the foot back to the tabletop. Alternate feet with each repetition.

- **Repetitions:** 10-12 per leg.

- **Purpose:** Strengthens the lower abdominals, improves coordination, and maintains stability in the core and arms.

17. Pilates Bar Supine Leg Extension

- **Starting Position:** Place your feet flat on the floor and bend your knees while lying on your back., holding the Pilates bar above your chest with arms extended.

- **Steps:** Extend one leg at a time towards the ceiling, pressing the sole of your foot against the middle of the Pilates bar. Gently press upwards against the bar to create slight resistance, then bend the knee to return to the starting position. Alternate legs.

- **Repetitions:** 8-10 per leg.

- **Purpose:** Enhances flexibility of the hamstrings, strengthens the quads, and engages the core, while the arms remain active.

18. Pilates Bar Mermaid Stretch

- **Starting Position:** Sit with legs folded to one side, creating a Z-shape. Hold the Pilates bar in both hands, extending it up over your head.

- **Steps:** Lean to the side opposite your legs, keeping the bar extended over your head, to feel a stretch along your side. Return to the center and switch sides to repeat the stretch.

- **Repetitions:** 5-8 per side.

- **Purpose:** Increases lateral flexibility of the spine, stretches the side muscles, and promotes mobility in the shoulders.

19. Pilates Bar Squat to Press

- **Starting Position:** Position your feet hip-width apart, holding the Pilates bar at your chest with both hands.

- **Steps:** Perform a squat by bending your knees and lowering your hips back as if sitting in a chair. As you return to standing, press the bar overhead, extending your arms fully. Lower the bar back to your chest as you squat down again.

- **Repetitions:** 10-15.

- **Purpose:** Integrates lower body strength work with upper body mobility, enhancing coordination, and engaging the core throughout the movement.

20. Pilates Bar Plie with Upright Row

- **Starting Position:** Stand with feet wider than hip-width apart, toes turned out. Hold the Pilates bar in front of you with both hands, arms extended downwards.

- **Steps:** Bend your knees to lower into a plie squat, keeping your back straight and knees aligned with your toes. As you lower, lift the Pilates bar towards your chest in an upright row, elbows leading the movement. Lower the bar as you straighten your legs to return to standing.

- **Repetitions:** 10-12.

- **Purpose:** Strengthens the inner thighs, glutes, and calves, while the upright row targets the shoulders and upper back, promoting posture and upper body strength.

21. Pilates Bar Roll-Ups

- **Starting Position:** Sit on the floor with legs extended straight in front of you and the Pilates bar in your hands, arms extended overhead.

- **Steps:** Slowly roll down onto your back, vertebra by vertebra, keeping the bar extended above your head. Then, slowly roll back up to a sitting position, leading with the bar and engaging your abdominal muscles to pull you up.

- **Repetitions:** 8-10.

- **Purpose:** Strengthens the core, particularly the abdominals, while promoting spinal flexibility and control.

22. Pilates Bar Hip Lifts

- **Starting Position:** Lay flat on your back with your knees bent and your feet resting on the ground, and the Pilates bar placed over your hips, holding it with both hands for stability.

- **Steps:** Press your feet into the floor to lift your hips towards the ceiling, squeezing your glutes at the top of the movement. Ensure the Pilates bar adds slight resistance by pressing down gently. Lower your hips back to the floor with control.

- **Repetitions:** 10-15.

- **Purpose:** Targets the glutes and hamstrings, strengthens the lower back, and engages the core, with the Pilates bar enhancing the engagement of the pelvic muscles.

23. Pilates Bar Standing Twist

- **Starting Position:** Position your feet hip-width apart, holding the Pilates bar horizontally in front of you at chest height, elbows bent.

- **Steps:** Engage your core and rotate your torso to one side, keeping your hips facing forward and moving the bar to the side as far as comfortable. Return to center and repeat on the opposite side.

- **Repetitions:** 10-12 per side.

- **Purpose:** Enhances core strength and flexibility, particularly focusing on the obliques, and improves rotational mobility.

24. Pilates Bar Arm and Leg Extension

- **Starting Position:** Get on all fours with the Pilates bar held in your hands, positioned directly under your shoulders.

- **Steps:** Extend one arm forward and the opposite leg back, keeping both parallel to the floor. Hold for a moment, then return to the starting position and switch sides.

- **Repetitions:** 8-10 per side.

- **Purpose:** Builds core stability and balance, strengthens the back, and engages the glutes and shoulders, promoting body coordination and control.

25. Pilates Bar Ankle Stretch and Strengthen

- **Starting Position:** Sit with legs extended in front of you and the Pilates bar resting on your lower legs, just above the ankles.

- **Steps:** Flex your feet, pressing against the bar to create resistance, then point your toes away from you, stretching the bar slightly forward. Move through flex and point with control.

- **Repetitions:** 10-15.

- **Purpose:** Increases ankle flexibility and strengthens the muscles around the lower leg and foot, improving mobility and supporting injury prevention.

26. Pilates Bar Front Raise

- **Starting Position:** Stand with your feet hip-width apart, holding the Pilates bar in front of you with both hands, palms facing down.

- **Steps:** Keeping your arms straight, lift the bar up to shoulder height, then lower it back down with control. Keep your core engaged and back straight throughout the movement.

- **Repetitions:** 10-12.

- **Purpose:** Strengthens the shoulders and upper back, improves posture, and engages the core muscles for stability.

27. Pilates Bar Overhead Triceps Extension

- **Starting Position:** Sit or Position your feet hip-width apart, holding the Pilates bar overhead with both hands, elbows pointing forward.

- **Steps:** Bend your elbows to lower the bar behind your head, keeping your upper arms stationary. Then, extend your arms to lift the bar back to the starting position.

- **Repetitions:** 10-15.

- **Purpose:** Targets the triceps, enhances arm strength, and maintains core engagement for balance and stability.

28. Pilates Bar Windmill

- **Starting Position:** Stand with your feet wider than shoulder-width apart, holding the Pilates bar horizontally with both hands overhead.

- **Steps:** Keeping your legs straight, hinge at your hips to lower the bar towards one foot, rotating your torso as you descend. Return to the starting position and repeat on the other side.

- **Repetitions:** 8-10 per side.

- **Purpose:** Increases hamstring flexibility, strengthens the obliques, and improves coordination and balance.

29. Pilates Bar Leg Pulls

- **Starting Position:** Start in a plank position with the Pilates bar placed under your hands on the floor.

- **Steps:** Lift one leg off the ground, keeping it straight, and pulse it upwards for a few seconds before lowering it back down. Repeat with the other leg.

- **Repetitions:** 8-10 per leg.

- **Purpose:** Strengthens the core, glutes, and lower back, improves balance, and enhances focus and body control.

30. Pilates Bar Side Leg Lifts

- **Starting Position:** Lie on one side with your body in a straight line, using one hand for head support. Place the Pilates bar along your top leg, holding it in place with your top hand.

- **Steps:** Lift your top leg towards the ceiling, pressing against the bar to add resistance, then lower it back down with control.

- **Repetitions:** 10-15 per side.

- **Purpose:** Targets the outer thighs and glutes, improves hip mobility, and engages the core for stabilization.

Special Motivational Quotes

1. "Strength does not come from physical capacity. It comes from an indomitable will to improve, grow, and transform your life, one Pilates bar workout at a time."

2. "Every movement in Pilates is a chance to find balance between body and mind. Embrace the journey, for each step forward is a step towards your best self."

3. "In the realm of Pilates, progress is not measured by the height of your bar, but by the depth of your commitment. Trust the process, and the transformation will follow."

4. "The power of Pilates is in its simplicity and precision. With each breath and movement, you are sculpting a stronger, more resilient version of yourself."

5. "Remember, the goal of Pilates is not to perfect each exercise but to perfect your understanding of your own strength and potential. Let the Pilates bar be your guide to unlocking the extraordinary within the ordinary."

Thank You Message

Thank you, dear readers, for embarking on this journey through the world of Pilates bar workouts for beginners. Your dedication to exploring new paths to health and wellness is commendable and inspiring. It is our hope that this guide has provided you with valuable insights, practical exercises, and the motivation to continue exploring the transformative power of Pilates. Remember, every effort you make towards bettering your physical and mental well-being is a step in the right direction. We are grateful for your commitment to self-improvement and for choosing this guide as a companion on your journey. May you continue to grow stronger, more flexible, and more balanced, both in body and mind. Here's to your health, happiness, and the endless possibilities that lie ahead. Thank you for allowing us to be a part of your Pilates journey.

CONCLUSION

Embarking on the journey of Pilates bar workouts as a beginner offers a unique opportunity to transform your physical health, enhance your mental well-being, and discover a deeper sense of body awareness. This guide has introduced a variety of exercises designed to cater to beginners, emphasizing the foundational principles of Pilates such as control, precision, and flow, all while incorporating the versatile Pilates bar. The exercises have been carefully selected to ensure a comprehensive approach to fitness, targeting core stability, flexibility, balance, and overall strength.

The beauty of Pilates bar workouts lies in their adaptability and focus on mind-body connection. As you progress through the exercises, you will likely notice improvements not just in your physical appearance, but in your posture, energy levels, and even in the ease with which you perform daily activities. The Pilates bar acts as a supportive tool, enhancing traditional Pilates exercises and making them accessible to beginners. Its use encourages proper alignment, increases resistance for muscle strengthening, and adds a creative twist to the Pilates practice.

Safety and mindfulness have been stressed throughout, with the acknowledgment that understanding one's own body is crucial in avoiding injury and achieving the best results. As with any fitness regimen, consistency is key. Regular practice will yield the most significant benefits, allowing the principles of Pilates to become second nature.

For beginners embarking on this journey, remember that Pilates is not just a series of exercises, but a path towards a healthier lifestyle. It teaches patience, awareness, and discipline. The inclusion of the Pilates bar enriches this practice, offering new challenges and ways to explore movement. Whether your goal is to improve physical fitness, recover from an injury, or find a moment of peace in a busy schedule, Pilates bar workouts provide a solid foundation upon which to build a stronger, more balanced self.

FITNESS

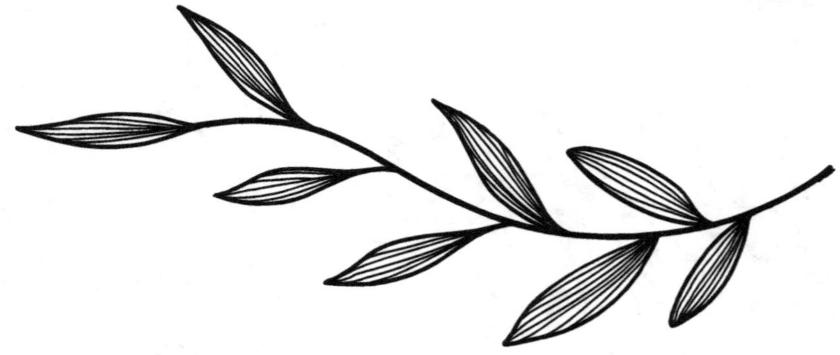

PLANNER

Fitness Planner

NAME:

DATE:

BREAKFAST

LUNCH

DINNER

SNACK

EXERCISE

SET

REP

NOTES

Fitness Planner

NAME: **DATE:**

BREAKFAST

LUNCH

DINNER

SNACK

EXERCISE

SET	REP	NOTES

Fitness Planner

NAME: **DATE:**

BREAKFAST

LUNCH

DINNER

SNACK

EXERCISE   SET   REP   NOTES

Fitness Planner

NAME: **DATE:**

BREAKFAST

LUNCH

DINNER

SNACK

EXERCISE

SET **REP** **NOTES**

Fitness Planner

NAME:

DATE:

BREAKFAST

LUNCH

DINNER

SNACK

EXERCISE

SET

REP

NOTES

Fitness Planner

NAME:

DATE:

BREAKFAST

LUNCH

DINNER

SNACK

EXERCISE

SET

REP

NOTES

Fitness Planner

NAME: **DATE:**

BREAKFAST

LUNCH

DINNER

SNACK

EXERCISE

SET   REP   NOTES

Fitness Planner

NAME:

DATE:

BREAKFAST

LUNCH

DINNER

SNACK

EXERCISE

EXERCISE	SET	REP	NOTES

Fitness Planner

NAME:

DATE:

BREAKFAST

LUNCH

DINNER

SNACK

EXERCISE

SET   REP   NOTES

Fitness Planner

NAME: **DATE:**

BREAKFAST

LUNCH

DINNER

SNACK

EXERCISE	SET	REP	NOTES

www.ingramcontent.com/pod-product-compliance
Lightning Source LLC
Chambersburg PA
CBHW070721260726
48660CB00007B/2679